AUTOIMMUNE

Protocol Juicing

COOKBOOK

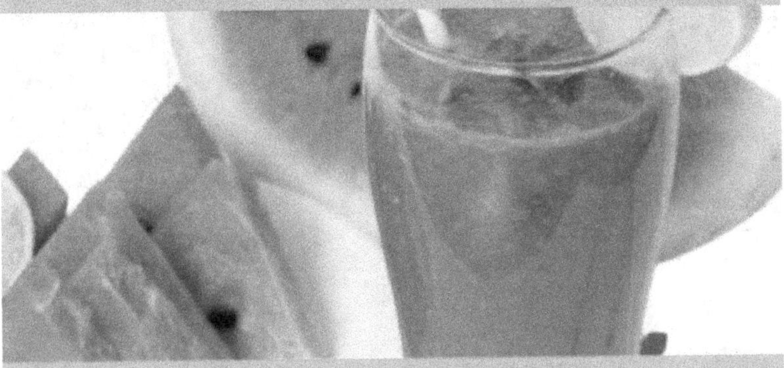

Easy Fruit Blends Nourish, Thrive With Anti-inflammatory Recipes For Gut Health, increased Energy And Weight Management.

Leona Butler

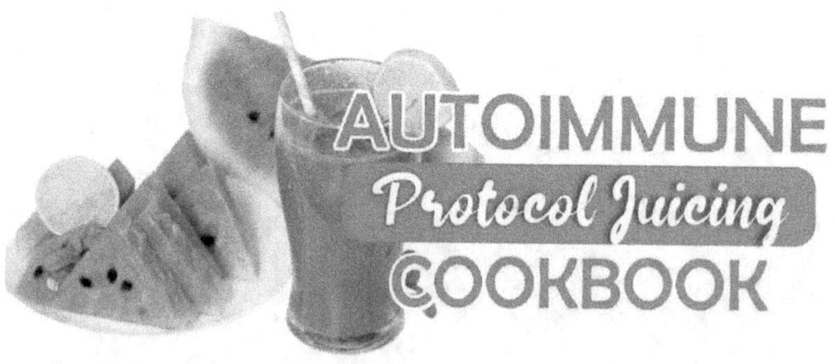
AUTOIMMUNE
Protocol Juicing
COOKBOOK

1. Familiarize Yourself: Begin by familiarizing yourself with the cookbook. Read the introduction, tips, and any guidelines provided about autoimmune protocol juicing.

2. Understand the Autoimmune Protocol (AIP): Understand the principles of the autoimmune protocol diet, which typically involves eliminating certain foods to reduce inflammation and support healing.

3. Gather Ingredients: Take note of the ingredients needed for the recipes you're interested in and make sure you have them on hand.

4. Follow Recipes: Follow the recipes in the cookbook carefully, paying attention to measurements and instructions.

5. Modify if Necessary: If you have specific dietary restrictions or preferences, feel free to modify the recipes accordingly while still adhering to the autoimmune protocol guidelines.

6. Experiment: Don't be afraid to experiment with different ingredient combinations or tweak the recipes to suit your taste preferences.

7. Use Fresh Ingredients: Opt for fresh, organic ingredients whenever possible to maximize the nutritional benefits of your juices.

8. Invest in a Good Juicer: Invest in a high-quality juicer to ensure that you're able to extract the most juice from your ingredients.

9. Stay Consistent: Incorporate juicing into your daily routine to reap the full benefits of the autoimmune protocol diet.

10. Listen to Your Body: Pay attention to how your body responds to the juices and adjust your recipes and consumption accordingly to support your health goals.

Table of Content

Introduction:

1. Understanding Autoimmune Diseases:

BENEFITS OF JUICING FOR AUTOIMMUNE HEALTH:

HOW AIP JUICING CAN SUPPORT HEALING:

2. Getting Started With Aip Juicing:

SELECTING THE RIGHT INGREDIENTS:

ESSENTIAL EQUIPMENT AND TOOLS:

TIPS FOR JUICING SUCCESS:

3. Smoothie Recipes

1. BERRY BLAST SMOOTHIE:

2. GREEN GODDESS SMOOTHIE:

3. TROPICAL TURMERIC SMOOTHIE:

4. CREAMY AVOCADO LIME SMOOTHIE:

5. BLUEBERRY KALE POWER SMOOTHIE:

6. MANGO GINGER TURMERIC SMOOTHIE:

7. PINEAPPLE CUCUMBER MINT SMOOTHIE:

8. CARROT CAKE SMOOTHIE:

9. CITRUS SUNSHINE SMOOTHIE:

10. CREAMY PEACH BASIL SMOOTHIE:

11. BEET BERRY BLISS SMOOTHIE:

12. PAPAYA KIWI DELIGHT SMOOTHIE:

13. CHERRY ALMOND SMOOTHIE:

14. CHOCOLATE MINT DREAM SMOOTHIE:

15. APPLE PIE SMOOTHIE:

4. Juicing Recipes

1. Carrot Ginger Zinger Juice:

2. Green Revitalizer Juice:

3. Citrus Beet Cleanse Juice:

4. Cucumber Mint Cooler Juice:

5. Pineapple Turmeric Elixir Juice:

6. Red Pepper Power Juice:

7. Sweet Potato Spice Juice:

8. Watermelon Basil Refresher Juice:

9. Berry Beet Blast Juice:

10. Mango Tango Juice:

11. Papaya Lime Quencher Juice:

12. Spinach Cucumber Cooler Juice

13. Orange Carrot Glow Juice

14. Pear Kiwi Kale Juice

15. Blueberry Basil Bliss Juice:

5. Bonus 1: Weeks Meal Planner

The Paperback Of This Version Has A Weeks Meal Planner

6. Conclusion

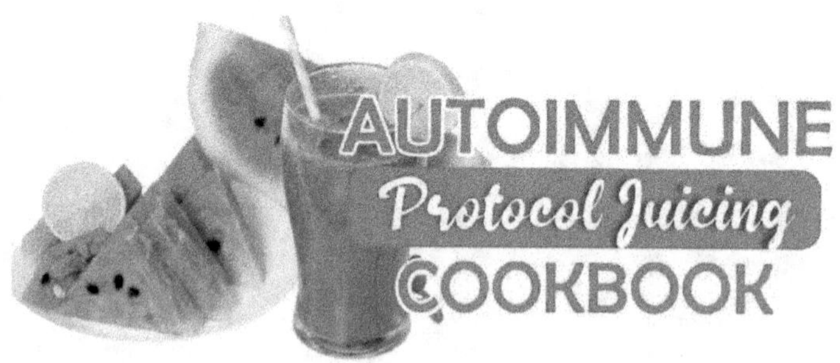

Introduction

Welcome to the Autoimmune Protocol Juicing Cookbook, where vibrant health meets delicious simplicity. Dive into a world of nutrient-rich juices that not only tantalize your taste buds but also support your body's natural healing process.

Inside, you'll discover a treasure trove of recipes designed to boost immunity, reduce inflammation, and promote overall wellness. Harness the power of nature's bounty with ingredients like leafy greens, turmeric, ginger, and berries, carefully selected for their anti-inflammatory properties and gut-healing benefits. Experience the rejuvenating effects of detoxification while staying hydrated and energized throughout your day.

Whether you're seeking weight management support, improved digestion, or glowing skin, these recipes offer a holistic approach to health and vitality. Empower yourself with the tools to thrive on the Autoimmune Protocol and embark on a journey towards optimal well-being, one delicious sip at a time."

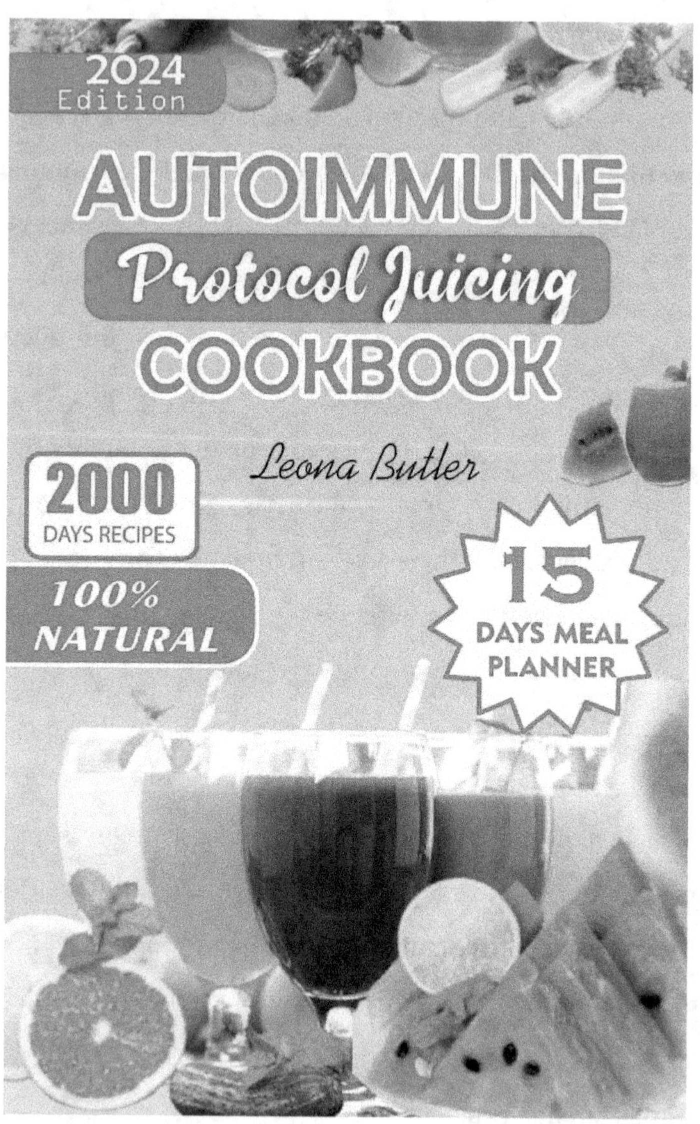

2024 Edition
AUTOIMMUNE
Protocol Juicing
COOKBOOK
Leona Butler
2000
DAYS RECIPES
100% NATURAL
15 DAYS MEAL PLANNER

1. Understanding Autoimmune Diseases

Autoimmune diseases occur when the immune system, which typically defends the body against pathogens, erroneously targets healthy cells, tissues, and organs. Conditions such as rheumatoid arthritis, lupus, multiple sclerosis, and celiac disease are examples of autoimmune disorders, each characterized by specific target tissues and symptoms. While the exact causes of autoimmune diseases remain elusive, factors such as genetics, environmental triggers, and dysregulation of the immune system are believed to play significant roles in their development.

Benefits of Juicing for Autoimmune Health:

Juicing, the process of extracting liquid from fruits, vegetables, and herbs, offers a concentrated source of essential nutrients, antioxidants, and phytochemicals. Incorporating freshly made juices into the diet can provide numerous benefits for individuals with autoimmune conditions:

1. Nutrient Density: Juicing allows for the consumption of a diverse range of nutrients in a form that is easily absorbed by the body. Vitamins, minerals, and antioxidants present in fruits and vegetables support immune function, reduce inflammation, and promote tissue repair, crucial aspects of managing autoimmune diseases.

2. Anti-Inflammatory Effects: Many fruits and vegetables used in juicing possess anti-inflammatory properties, helping to mitigate the chronic inflammation characteristic of autoimmune disorders. Compounds such as flavonoids, carotenoids, and polyphenols found in colorful produce exhibit potent anti-inflammatory effects, offering relief from symptoms and potentially slowing disease progression.

3. Gut Health Support: The gut plays a pivotal role in the development and modulation of the immune system, making gut health a focal point in managing autoimmune diseases. Juicing with gut-friendly ingredients such as ginger, turmeric, and probiotic-rich foods can help restore microbial balance, strengthen the gut barrier, and alleviate gastrointestinal symptoms commonly associated with autoimmune conditions.

4. Detoxification: Juicing can aid the body's natural detoxification processes by providing an influx of nutrients that support liver function and cellular repair. By reducing the burden of toxins and promoting elimination, juicing may alleviate symptoms exacerbated by environmental toxins and promote overall well-being.

How AIP Juicing Can Support Healing:

The Autoimmune Protocol (AIP) is a dietary approach specifically designed to address autoimmune diseases by eliminating potentially inflammatory foods and prioritizing nutrient-dense, anti-inflammatory options. When integrated with juicing, the AIP becomes a powerful tool for supporting healing and managing symptoms:

1. Selective Ingredient Choices: AIP-friendly juicing focuses on ingredients permitted within the protocol, such as leafy greens, cruciferous vegetables, low-glycemic fruits, and healing herbs. By avoiding common trigger foods like grains, dairy, nightshades, and processed sugars, AIP juicing minimizes potential immune reactions and promotes healing from within.

2. Targeted Nutrient Delivery: AIP juicing allows for precise nutrient delivery tailored to the specific needs of individuals with autoimmune diseases. Ingredients rich in vitamin C, vitamin A, zinc, and omega-3 fatty acids support immune modulation, tissue repair, and the restoration of healthy cellular function, addressing underlying imbalances contributing to autoimmune pathogenesis.

3. Enhanced Symptom Management: By combining the therapeutic principles of the AIP with the nutritional benefits of juicing, individuals can experience improved symptom management and quality of life. Reductions in pain, fatigue, inflammation, and autoimmune flares are commonly reported outcomes, empowering individuals to take an active role in their health and well-being.

2. Getting Started with AIP Juicing

The Autoimmune Protocol (AIP) is a dietary approach designed to reduce inflammation and support those with autoimmune conditions. Juicing on the AIP involves extracting nutrient-rich juices from fruits and vegetables to provide concentrated sources of vitamins and minerals. Before diving into juicing, it's essential to understand the principles behind AIP and how to incorporate it into your lifestyle.

Selecting the Right Ingredients

Choosing the right ingredients is crucial when juicing on the AIP. Focus on organic, fresh fruits, and vegetables that are compliant with the AIP guidelines. This typically includes nutrient-dense options like leafy greens (kale, spinach), low-sugar fruits (berries, green apples), and non-nightshade vegetables (carrots, cucumbers). Avoid ingredients such as tomatoes, peppers, and eggplants, which are not AIP-friendly due to their potential to trigger inflammation.

Essential Equipment and Tools

Investing in the right equipment is key to successful juicing on the AIP. A high-quality juicer is essential for efficiently extracting juice from fruits and vegetables while preserving their nutritional value. Look for a masticating or cold-press juicer, as they tend to retain more nutrients compared to centrifugal juicers. Additionally, you'll need a sharp knife for preparing produce, a cutting board, and a pitcher or container to collect the juice.

Tips for Juicing Success

1. Plan Ahead: Take time to plan your juice recipes and ensure you have an adequate supply of fresh produce on hand. Planning ahead can help you stay consistent with your juicing routine.

2. Start Simple: Begin with straightforward juice combinations and gradually experiment with different ingredients to find what works best for your taste preferences and nutritional needs.

3. Rotate Ingredients: Rotate your ingredients regularly to ensure you're getting a variety of nutrients and to prevent developing sensitivities to specific foods.

4. Include Healthy Fats: Incorporate healthy fats into your juices by adding ingredients like avocado or coconut oil. Fats help improve nutrient absorption and provide satiety.

5. Mindful Consumption: While juicing can be a convenient way to increase your intake of fruits and vegetables, it's essential to consume juices mindfully and not solely rely on them for nutrition. Whole foods should still form the foundation of your AIP diet.

6. Stay Hydrated: In addition to juicing, remember to drink plenty of water throughout the day to stay hydrated and support overall health and digestion.

7. Listen to Your Body: Pay attention to how your body responds to different ingredients and adjust your juicing recipes accordingly. Everyone's dietary needs and tolerances are unique, so customize your approach based on what works best for you.

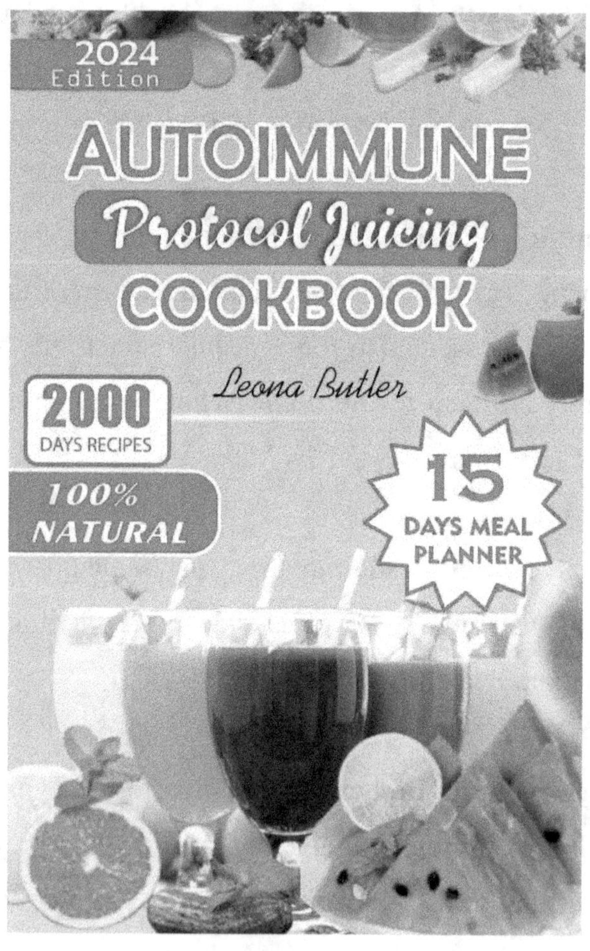

3. Smoothie Recipes

1. Berry Blast Smoothie:

Ingredients:

- 1 cup mixed berries (strawberries, blueberries, raspberries)
- 1 banana
- 1/2 cup Greek yogurt
- 1/2 cup almond milk
- 1 tablespoon honey (optional) Ice cubes (optional)

Preparation:

1. Add all the ingredients into a blender.
2. Blend until smooth and creamy.
3. Serve immediately.

Nutritional Value:

- Calories: Approximately 200-250 calories per serving

- Rich in antioxidants, vitamin C, potassium, and probiotics from the yogurt.

Preparation time: 5 minutes

2. Green Goddess Smoothie

Ingredients:

- 2 cups spinach leaves
- 1 ripe avocado
- 1/2 cucumber, peeled and chopped
- 1/2 cup pineapple chunks
- 1/2 cup coconut water
- Juice of 1 lime
- Ice cubes (optional)

Preparation:

1. Place all the ingredients in a blender.
2. Blend until smooth and creamy.
3. Adjust the consistency by adding more coconut water as needed.

Serve immediately.

Nutritional Value:

- Calories: Approximately 250-300 calories per serving High in fiber, healthy fats, potassium, vitamin C, and electrolytes.

Preparation time: 5 minutes

3. Tropical Turmeric Smoothie

Ingredients:

- 1 cup frozen mango chunks
- 1/2 cup frozen pineapple chunks
- 1 ripe banana
- 1 teaspoon turmeric powder 1/2 teaspoon ginger powder
- 1 cup coconut milk
- 1 tablespoon honey (optional) Ice cubes (optional)

Preparation:

1. Place all ingredients into a blender.
2. Blend until smooth and creamy.

3. Taste and adjust sweetness with honey if desired.

4. Serve immediately.

Nutritional Value:

- Calories: Approximately 250-300 calories per serving

- High in vitamin C, fiber, antioxidants, and anti-inflammatory properties from turmeric.

Preparation time: 5 minutes

4. Creamy Avocado Lime Smoothie

Ingredients:

- 1 ripe avocado

- Juice of 2 limes

- 1 cup spinach leaves

- 1/2 cup plain Greek yogurt

- 1/2 cup almond milk

- 1 tablespoon honey (optional) Ice cubes (optional)

Preparation:

- Combine all ingredients in a blender.

- Blend until smooth and creamy.

- Taste and add honey as needed to adjust the sweetness.

- Serve immediately.

Nutritional Value:

- Calories: Approximately 200-250 calories per serving Rich in healthy fats, vitamin C, potassium, and protein from yogurt.

Preparation time: 5 minutes

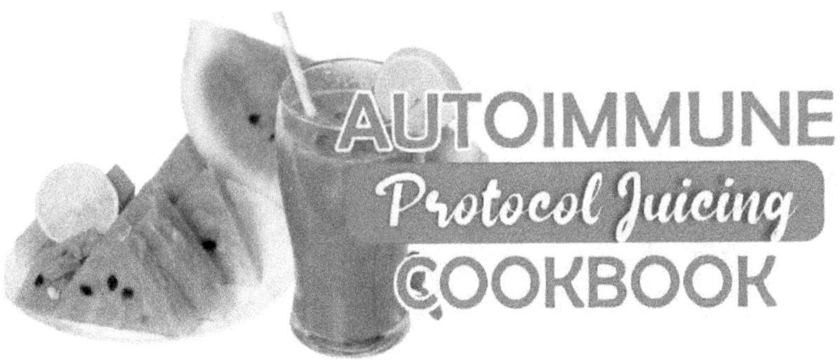

Ingredients:

- 1 cup fresh or frozen blueberries
- 1 cup chopped kale leaves
- 1 banana
- 1 tablespoon chia seeds
- 1 cup almond milk
- 1 tablespoon honey or maple syrup (optional)

Preparation:

- Place all ingredients in a blender.
- Blend until smooth.
- Serve immediately.

Nutritional Value (approximate per serving):

- Calories: 250
- Protein: 5g
- Fat: 7g
- Carbohydrates: 45g
- Fiber: 10g

Ingredients:

- 1 cup chopped mango
- 1 tablespoon grated ginger
- 1 teaspoon ground turmeric
- 1 cup coconut water
- 1/2 cup Greek yogurt
- 1 tablespoon honey or agave syrup (optional)

Preparation:

1. Combine all ingredients in a blender.
2. Blend until smooth.
3. Pour into glasses and serve immediately.

Nutritional Value (approximate per serving):

- Calories: 200
- Protein: 7g
- Fat: 1g
- Carbohydrates: 40g
- Fiber: 5g

Ingredients:

- 1 cup chopped pineapple
- 1/2 cup chopped cucumber
- 1/4 cup fresh mint leaves
- Juice of 1 lime
- 1 cup coconut water Ice cubes (optional)

Preparation:

1. Put all ingredients in a blender.
2. Blend until smooth.
3. Add ice cubes if desired and blend again.
4. Pour into glasses and serve immediately.

Nutritional Value (approximate per serving):

- Calories: 120
- Protein: 2g
- Fat: 0.5g
- Carbohydrates: 30g
- Fiber: 4g

Ingredients:

- 1 cup chopped carrots
- 1 banana
- 1/4 cup rolled oats
- 1/2 teaspoon ground cinnamon
- 1/4 teaspoon ground nutmeg
- 1 cup almond milk
- 1 tablespoon honey or maple syrup (optional) Ice cubes (optional)

Preparation:

1. Combine all ingredients in a blender.
2. Blend until smooth.
3. Add ice cubes if desired and blend again.
4. Pour into glasses and serve immediately.

Nutritional Value (approximate per serving):

- Calories: 220

- Protein: 5g

- Fat: 3g

- Carbohydrates: 45g

- Fiber: 7g

9. Citrus Sunshine Smoothie

Ingredients:

- 1 orange, peeled and segmented

- 1/2 grapefruit, peeled and segmented

- 1 banana, frozen

- 1/2 cup Greek yogurt

- 1/2 cup almond milk

- 1 tablespoon honey (optional) Ice cubes (optional)

Preparation:

1. Place the orange segments, grapefruit segments, frozen banana, Greek yogurt, almond milk, and honey (if using) in a blender.
2. Blend until smooth and creamy.
3. If required, add more ice cubes and mix until smooth.
4. Pour into glasses and serve immediately.

Nutritional Value:

- Calories: Approximately 250
- Protein: 10g
- Fat: 3g
- Carbohydrates: 50g
- Fiber: 7g
- Vitamin C: 100% of daily recommended intake

Ingredients:

- 2 ripe peaches, pitted and sliced
- 1/2 cup plain yogurt
- 1/4 cup fresh basil leaves
- 1/2 cup almond milk
- 1 tablespoon honey or maple syrup (optional) Ice cubes (optional)

Preparation:

1. Place the sliced peaches, plain yogurt, fresh basil leaves, almond milk, and honey or maple syrup (if using) in a blender.
2. Blend until smooth and creamy.
3. Add ice cubes if desired and blend again until smooth.
4. Pour into glasses and garnish with a fresh basil leaf, if desired.
5. Serve immediately.

Nutritional Value:

- Calories: Approximately 200
- Protein: 8g
- Fat: 2g
- Carbohydrates: 40g
- Fiber: 5g
- Vitamin A: 30% of daily recommended intake Vitamin C: 70% of daily recommended intake Enjoy your refreshing smoothies!

11. Beet Berry Bliss Smoothie

Ingredients:

- 1 small beet, peeled and diced
- 1 cup mixed berries (strawberries, blueberries, raspberries)
- 1 banana, peeled and sliced
- 1/2 cup Greek yogurt
- 1 tablespoon honey or maple syrup 1 cup almond milk or any other preferred milk

Preparation:

1. Place all the ingredients into a blender.

2. Blend until smooth and creamy.

3. Serve immediately and enjoy!

Nutritional Value:

- Calories: Approximately 220

- Protein: 8g

- Fat: 4g

- Carbohydrates: 40g

- Fiber: 7g

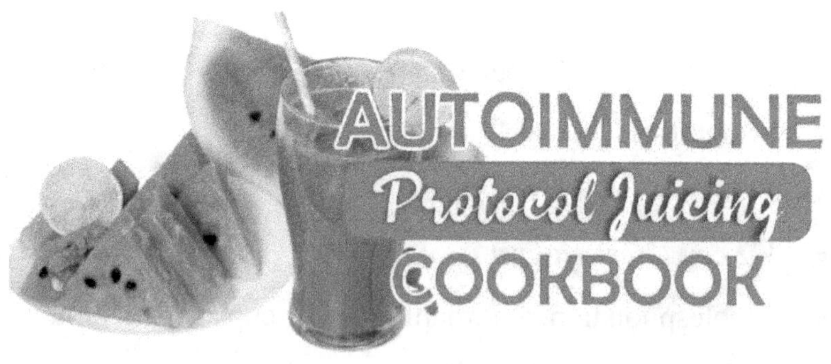

12. Papaya Kiwi Delight Smoothie

Ingredients:

- cup diced papaya
- kiwis, peeled and sliced
- 1/2 cup plain yogurt
- 1 tablespoon honey or agave syrup
- 1/2 cup coconut water or pineapple juice Ice cubes (optional)

Preparation:

1. Add all the ingredients to a blender.
2. Blend until smooth and creamy.
3. If desired, add ice cubes and blend again for a colder texture.
4. Pour into glasses and serve chilled.

Nutritional Value:

- Calories: Approximately 200
- Protein: 4g
- Fat: 2g
- Carbohydrates: 45g
- Fiber: 7g

13. Cherry Almond Smoothie

Ingredients:

- 1 cup frozen cherries
- 1/4 cup almonds
- 1 ripe banana
- 1 cup spinach leaves
- 1 tablespoon almond butter
- 1 cup almond milk
- 1 teaspoon vanilla extract Ice cubes (optional)

Preparation:

1. Combine all ingredients in a blender.

2. Blend until smooth and creamy.

3. Add ice cubes if a colder consistency is desired.

4. Pour into glasses and serve immediately.

Nutritional Value:

*   Calories: Approximately 280

*   Protein: 8g

*   Fat: 12g

*   Carbohydrates: 38g

*   Fiber: 9g

Enjoy these nutritious and delicious smoothies!

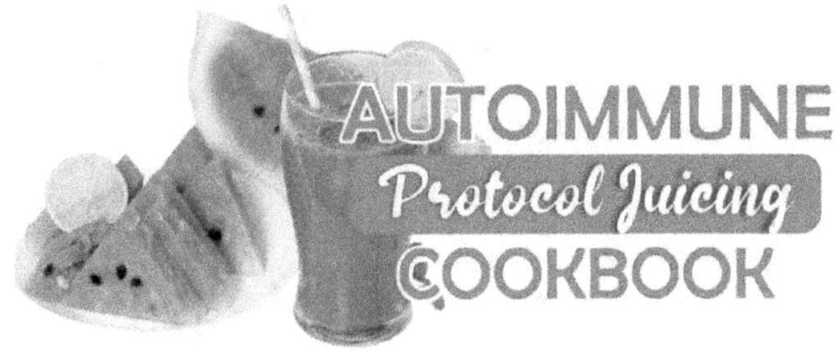

Ingredients:

- 1 cup almond milk
- 1 ripe banana
- 1 tablespoon cocoa powder·
- 1 tablespoon honey or maple syrup
- 1/2 teaspoon peppermint extract
- 1 handful spinach leaves
- 1/2 cup ice cubes

Preparation:

1. In a blender, combine almond milk, banana, cocoa powder, honey or maple syrup, peppermint extract, spinach leaves, and ice cubes.
2. Blend until smooth and creamy.
3. Pour into a glass and serve immediately.

Nutritional Value (per serving):

- Calories: 180
- Protein: 3g
- Fat: 3g
- Carbohydrates: 38g
- Fiber: 5g
- Sugar: 22g
- Vitamin A: 35% DV
- Vitamin C: 30% DV
- Calcium: 25% DV
- Iron: 10% DV

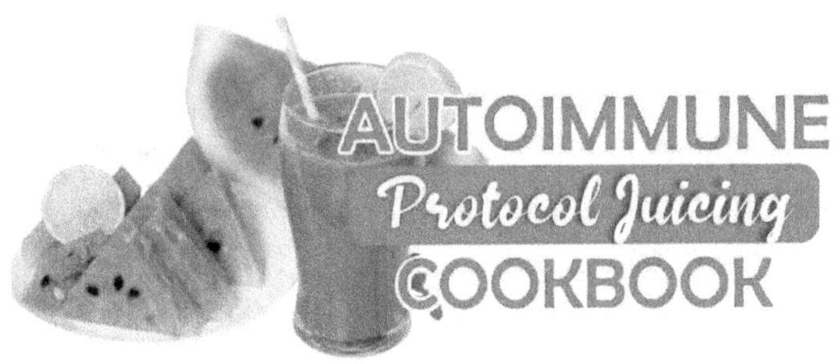

15. Apple Pie Smoothie

Ingredients:

- 1 cup unsweetened applesauce
- 1/2 cup plain Greek yogurt
- 1/2 cup almond milk
- 1 small apple, cored and chopped
- 1 tablespoon honey or maple syrup
- 1/2 teaspoon ground cinnamon
- 1/4 teaspoon ground nutmeg
- 1/4 teaspoon vanilla extract
- 1/2 cup ice cubes

Preparation:

1. In a blender, combine unsweetened applesauce, Greek yogurt, almond milk, chopped apple, honey or maple syrup, ground cinnamon, ground nutmeg, vanilla extract, and ice cubes.
2. Blend until smooth and creamy.
3. Pour into a glass and sprinkle with additional cinnamon if desired. Serve immediately.

Nutritional Value (per serving):

- Calories: 160

- Protein: 6g

- Fat: 2g

- Carbohydrates: 32g

- Fiber: 5g

- Sugar: 22g

- Vitamin A: 2% DV

- Vitamin C: 10% DV

- Calcium: 15% DV

- Iron: 4% DV

Enjoy your delicious and nutritious smoothies!

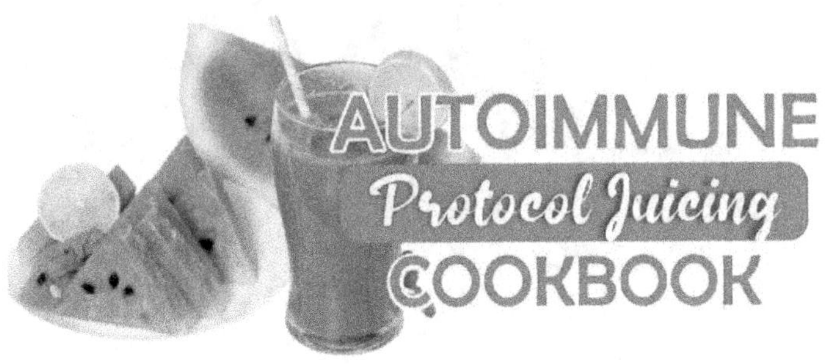

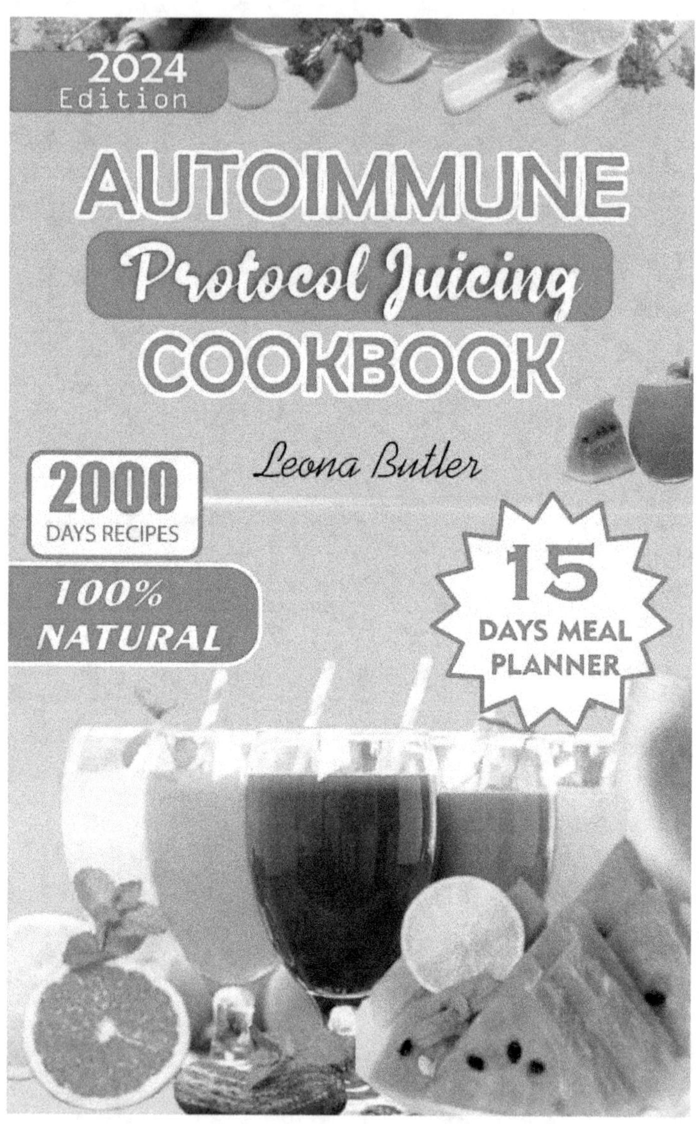

2024 Edition
AUTOIMMUNE
Protocol Juicing
COOKBOOK
Leona Butler
2000
DAYS RECIPES
100% NATURAL
15
DAYS MEAL
PLANNER

4. Juicing Recipes

1. Carrot Ginger Zinger Juice:

Ingredients:

- 4 large carrots, peeled and chopped
- 1-inch piece of ginger, peeled
- 1 medium-sized apple, cored and chopped
- 1 lemon, peeled
- 1 tablespoon honey (optional)
- 1 cup water (adjust for desired consistency)

Preparation:
- Place all ingredients in a juicer.
- Juice until smooth.
- If desired, add honey to sweeten.
- Serve over ice.

Nutritional Value (per serving):
- Calories: ~120
- Carbohydrates: ~28g

- Fiber: ~5g

- Protein: ~2g

- Fat: ~1g

2. Green Revitalizer Juice

Ingredients:

- 2 cups spinach

- cucumber, peeled and chopped

- stalks celery, chopped

- 1 green apple, cored and chopped

- 1/2 lemon, peeled

- 1-inch piece of ginger, peeled 1 cup water (adjust for desired consistency)

Preparation:

- Add all ingredients to a juicer.

- Juice until well blended.

- Pour into a glass and serve immediately.

Nutritional Value (per serving):

- Calories: ~80
- Carbohydrates: ~20g
- Fiber: ~5g
- Protein: ~3g
- Fat: ~1g

3. Citrus Beet Cleanse Juice

Ingredients:

- large beet, peeled and chopped
- oranges, peeled
- 1 large carrot, peeled and chopped
- 1-inch piece of ginger, peeled
- 1/2 lemon, peeled
- 1 cup water (adjust for desired consistency)

Preparation:

1. Place all ingredients in a juicer.

2. Juice until smooth.

3. Adjust water as needed for consistency.

4. Serve immediately over ice.

Nutritional Value (per serving):

- Calories: ~110

- Carbohydrates: ~25g

- Fiber: ~6g

- Protein: ~3g

- Fat: ~1g

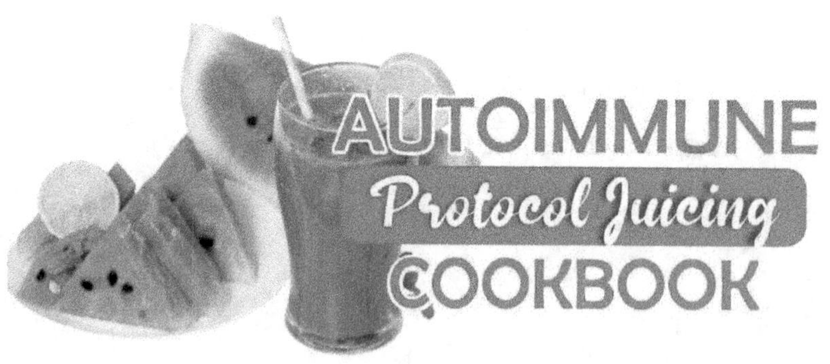

4. Cucumber Mint Cooler Juice

Ingredients:

- 2 medium cucumbers, peeled and chopped
- 1/4 cup fresh mint leaves
- 1/2 lime, juiced
- 1 cup cold water Ice cubes (optional)

Preparation:

1. In a blender, combine the chopped cucumbers, fresh mint leaves, lime juice, and cold water.
2. Blend until smooth.
3. To remove the pulp, strain the mixture through a fine-mesh screen.
4. Serve over ice cubes if desired.

Nutritional Value:

Cucumbers are a low-calorie food high in vitamin K and potassium. Mint leaves can help digestion and add a refreshing flavor.

5. Pineapple Turmeric Elixir Juice

Ingredients:

- 2 cups fresh pineapple chunks
- 1 teaspoon ground turmeric 1/2 teaspoon ground ginger
- 1 tablespoon honey (optional)
- 1 cup coconut water

Preparation:

1. In a blender, combine the fresh pineapple chunks, ground turmeric, ground ginger, honey (if using), and coconut water.
2. Blend until smooth.
3. Taste and adjust sweetness as needed by adding additional honey.
4. Serve chilled.

6. Red Pepper Power Juice:

Ingredients:

- Two large red bell peppers, seeded and sliced.

- 2 medium carrots, peeled and chopped

- 1 medium tomato, chopped

- 1/2 lemon, juiced

- 1/4 teaspoon cayenne pepper (optional)

- 1 cup cold water

Preparation:

1. In a blender, combine the chopped red bell peppers, carrots, tomato, lemon juice, cayenne pepper (if using), and cold water.

2. Blend until smooth.

3. To remove the pulp, strain the mixture through a fine-mesh screen.

4. Serve chilled or over ice cubes.

7. Sweet Potato Spice Juice:

Ingredients:

- 2 medium sweet potatoes, peeled and chopped
- 1 apple, cored and chopped
- 1 teaspoon ground cinnamon
- 1/2 teaspoon ground nutmeg
- 1/4 teaspoon ground ginger 1 cup water or coconut water

Preparation:

1. Place all ingredients in a blender.
2. Blend until smooth.
3. If desired, strain the juice to remove any pulp.
4. Serve immediately.

Nutritional Value (per serving):
- Calories: 180
- Carbohydrates: 45g
- Fiber: 8g
- Sugars: 20g , Protein: 3g

Ingredients:

- 4 cups cubed seedless watermelon
- 1/4 cup fresh basil leaves
- 1 tablespoon lime juice
- 1 cup ice cubes

Preparation:

1. In a blender, combine watermelon, basil leaves, lime juice, and ice cubes.
2. Blend until smooth.
3. Pour into glasses and garnish with additional basil leaves or lime slices if desired.
4. Serve immediately.

Nutritional Value (per serving)

- Calories: 80
- Carbohydrates: 20g
- Fiber: 1g
- Sugars: 16g
- Protein: 1g

Ingredients:

- 1 medium beet, peeled and chopped
- 1 cup mixed berries (such as strawberries, blueberries, and raspberries).
- 1/2 cup spinach leaves
- 1 tablespoon honey or maple syrup (optional)
- 1 cup water or coconut water

Preparation:

1. Place all ingredients in a blender.
2. Blend until smooth.
3. If desired, add honey or maple syrup to modify the sweetness.

Nutritional Value (per serving):

- Calories: 100
- Carbohydrates: 25g
- Fiber: 5g
- Sugars: 18g
- Protein: 2g

10. Mango Tango Juice

Ingredients:

- 2 ripe mangoes, peeled and chopped
- 1 orange, peeled and segmented
- 1/2 cup pineapple chunks
- 1/2 cup water or coconut water
- Ice cubes (optional)

Preparation:

1. Combine all the ingredients in a blender.
2. Blend until smooth.
3. If required, add more ice cubes and mix until smooth.
4. Pour into glasses and serve chilled.

Nutritional Value (per serving):

- Calories: Approximately 150
- Carbohydrates: Approximately 38g
- Fiber: Approximately 5g
- Vitamin C: Approximately 100% of daily value

11. Papaya Lime Quencher Juice

Ingredients:

- 1 ripe papaya, peeled, seeded, and chopped
- Juice of 2 limes
- 1 tablespoon honey or agave syrup
- 1/2 cup cold water
- Ice cubes (optional)
- Fresh mint leaves for garnish (optional)

Preparation:

1. Place the chopped papaya, lime juice, honey or agave syrup, and cold water in a blender.
2. Blend until smooth.
3. Taste and adjust sweetness if needed by adding more honey or agave syrup.
4. If required, add more ice cubes and mix until smooth.
5. Pour into glasses, garnish with fresh mint leaves, and serve chilled.

Nutritional Value (per serving):

- Calories: Approximately 120

- Carbohydrates: Approximately 30g

- Fiber: Approximately 4g

- Vitamin A: Approximately 150% of daily value Vitamin
  C: Approximately 100% of daily value

12. Spinach Cucumber Cooler Juice

Ingredients:

- 2 cups fresh spinach leaves

- 1 cucumber, peeled and chopped

- 1 green apple, cored and chopped

- 1/2 lemon, juiced

- 1/2 cup cold water

- Ice cubes (optional)

- Fresh parsley for garnish (optional)

Preparation:

1. Place the spinach leaves, chopped cucumber, chopped green apple, lemon juice, and cold water in a blender.

2. Blend until smooth.

3. If required, add more ice cubes and mix until smooth.

4. Pour into glasses, garnish with fresh parsley, and serve chilled.

Nutritional Value (per serving):

- Calories: Approximately 80

- Carbohydrates: Approximately 20g

- Fiber: Approximately 6g

- Vitamin A: Approximately 200% of daily value Vitamin C: Approximately 80% of daily value Enjoy your refreshing and nutritious juices!

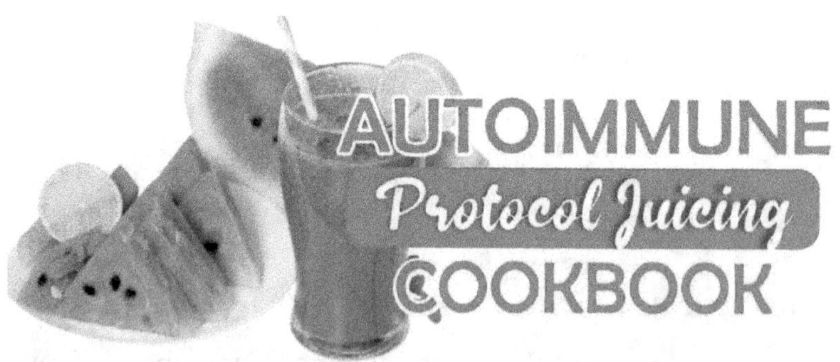

13. Orange Carrot Glow Juice

Ingredients:

- 2 large oranges, peeled and segmented
- 4 medium carrots, washed and trimmed
- 1 inch piece of ginger, peeled
- 1/2 lemon, peeled
- 1/4 cup water (optional, for consistency)

Preparation:

1. Place all ingredients into a juicer.
2. Process until smooth.
3. If desired, add water to adjust consistency.
4. Serve immediately and enjoy!

Nutritional Value (per serving):

- Calories: 120
- Total Fat: 0.5g
- Carbohydrates: 28g
- Fiber: 6g
- Sugars: 18g
- Protein: 2g

Ingredients:

- 2 ripe pears, cored and chopped
- 2 kiwis, peeled and chopped
- 2 cups kale leaves, washed and stems removed
- 1/2 cucumber, peeled and chopped
- 1/2 lemon, peeled
- 1/4 cup water (optional, for consistency)

Preparation:

1. Put all ingredients into a juicer.
2. Process until well combined and smooth.
3. Adjust consistency with water if needed.
4. Serve immediately and enjoy!

Nutritional Value (per serving):

- Calories: 150
- Total Fat: 0.5g
- Carbohydrates: 36g
- Fiber: 10g
- Sugars: 20g Protein: 4g

15. Blueberry Basil Bliss Juice:

Ingredients:

- 2 cups blueberries, fresh or frozen
- cup basil leaves, packed
- medium apples, cored and chopped
- 1/2 cucumber, peeled and chopped
- 1/2 lemon, peeled
- 1/4 cup water (optional, for consistency)

Preparation:

1. Combine all ingredients in a juicer.
2. Process until smooth.
3. Add water if needed to adjust consistency.
4. Serve immediately and enjoy!

Nutritional Value (per serving):

- Calories: 180
- Total Fat: 1g
- Carbohydrates: 44g
- Fiber: 10g
- Sugars: 28g

Protein: 3g

These juices are not only delicious but also packed with essential vitamins, minerals, and antioxidants for a healthy glow!

5. BONUS 1: weeks meal planner

The Paperback of This Version Has a Weeks Meal Planner

MY WEEKLY MEAL PLANNER

Date

	Breakfast	Lunch	Dinner
MON			
TUE			
WED			
THU			
FRI			
SAT			
SUN			

SHOPPING LIST:

TO DO LIST

NOTES AND TIPS

5. Conclusion

In conclusion, this Autoimmune Protocol (AIP) juicing cookbook offers a comprehensive array of delicious and nutritious recipes tailored to support those managing autoimmune conditions.

By incorporating nutrient-dense ingredients and eliminating potential triggers, this cookbook empowers individuals to take control of their health and well-being. From vibrant fruit blends to antioxidant-rich vegetable concoctions, each recipe is thoughtfully crafted to not only satisfy the palate but also promote healing from within. Embracing the AIP diet through juicing not only provides a flavorful journey but also fosters a deeper connection with one's body and its needs.

As you embark on this transformative culinary adventure, remember that every sip is a step towards vitality and resilience. Let the rejuvenating power of these juices inspire you to embrace and adapt to the AIP lifestyle, nurturing your body, mind, and spirit for a vibrant and fulfilling life ahead.

Thank you for immersing yourself in the pages of our Autoimmune Protocol (AIP) juicing cookbook. Your dedication to exploring and embracing the healing potential of nutrient-rich ingredients is truly inspiring. By choosing to prioritize your health and well-being, you're embarking on a journey towards vitality and resilience.

We're deeply grateful for your trust in our recipes and guidance as you navigate the complexities of managing autoimmune conditions. Your commitment to self-care is a powerful reminder of the importance of nurturing oneself from the inside out.

As you embark on this culinary adventure, know that you're not alone. Our heartfelt gratitude goes out to you for joining us on this journey towards better health and a brighter future. Here's to vibrant health, delicious flavors, and a life filled with wellness. Thank you for being a part of our community.

MY WEEKLY MEAL PLANNER

Date

	Breakfast	Lunch	Dinner
MON			
TUE			
WED			
THU			
FRI			
SAT			
SUN			

SHOPPING LIST:

To Do List

NOTES
AND TIPS

MY WEEKLY MEAL PLANNER

Date

	Breakfast	Lunch	Dinner
MON			
TUE			
WED			
THU			
FRI			
SAT			
SUN			

SHOPPING LIST:

To Do List

● ·
· · · · · · · · · · · · · · · · ·
· · · · · · · · · · · · · · · · ·
● ·
· · · · · · · · · · · · · · · · ·
· · · · · · · · · · · · · · · · ·
● ·
· · · · · · · · · · · · · · · · ·

● ·

NOTES
AND TIPS

MY WEEKLY MEAL PLANNER

Date

	Breakfast	Lunch	Dinner
MON			
TUE			
WED			
THU			
FRI			
SAT			
SUN			

SHOPPING LIST:

-
-
-
-

TO DO LIST

NOTES
AND TIPS

MY WEEKLY MEAL PLANNER

Date

	Breakfast	Lunch	Dinner
MON			
TUE			
WED			
THU			
FRI			
SAT			
SUN			

SHOPPING LIST:

To Do List

-
-
-
-

NOTES AND TIPS

MY WEEKLY MEAL PLANNER

Date

	Breakfast	Lunch	Dinner
Mon			
Tue			
Wed			
Thu			
Fri			
Sat			
Sun			

SHOPPING LIST:

To Do List

- ●
- ●
- ●
- ●

Notes
And Tips

MY WEEKLY MEAL PLANNER

Date

	Breakfast	Lunch	Dinner
MON			
TUE			
WED			
THU			
FRI			
SAT			
SUN			

SHOPPING LIST:

- ....
- ....
- ....
- ....

TO DO LIST

....
....
....
....
....

NOTES
AND TIPS

MY WEEKLY MEAL PLANNER

Date

	Breakfast	Lunch	Dinner
MON			
TUE			
WED			
THU			
FRI			
SAT			
SUN			

SHOPPING LIST:

To Do List

-
-
-
-

NOTES
AND TIPS

MY WEEKLY MEAL PLANNER

Date

	Breakfast	Lunch	Dinner
Mon			
Tue			
Wed			
Thu			
Fri			
Sat			
Sun			

SHOPPING LIST:

To Do List

Notes
And Tips

MY WEEKLY MEAL PLANNER

Date

	Breakfast	Lunch	Dinner
MON			
TUE			
WED			
THU			
FRI			
SAT			
SUN			

SHOPPING LIST:

To Do List

-
-
-
-

NOTES
AND TIPS

MY WEEKLY MEAL PLANNER

Date

	Breakfast	Lunch	Dinner
MON			
TUE			
WED			
THU			
FRI			
SAT			
SUN			

SHOPPING LIST:

To Do List

NOTES AND TIPS

MY WEEKLY MEAL PLANNER

Date

	Breakfast	Lunch	Dinner
MON			
TUE			
WED			
THU			
FRI			
SAT			
SUN			

SHOPPING LIST:

- ....
- ....
- ....
- ....

TO DO LIST

....
....
....
....
....

NOTES AND TIPS

MY WEEKLY MEAL PLANNER

Date

	Breakfast	Lunch	Dinner
MON			
TUE			
WED			
THU			
FRI			
SAT			
SUN			

SHOPPING LIST:

To Do List

-
-
-
-

NOTES
AND TIPS

MY WEEKLY MEAL PLANNER

Date

	Breakfast	Lunch	Dinner
MON			
TUE			
WED			
THU			
FRI			
SAT			
SUN			

SHOPPING LIST:

To Do List

NOTES AND TIPS

MY WEEKLY MEAL PLANNER

Date

	Breakfast	Lunch	Dinner
MON			
TUE			
WED			
THU			
FRI			
SAT			
SUN			

SHOPPING LIST:

TO DO LIST

NOTES
AND TIPS